Dayana Bra Vera
Zulma Díaz Hernández
Barbara Rodríguez de León

# Reversible acute serous transient reversible pulpitis

Dayana Bra Vera
Zulma Díaz Hernández
Barbara Rodríguez de León

# Reversible acute serous transient reversible pulpitis

## Evolution of treatment with eugenol as a pulp sedative up to 96 hours

ScienciaScripts

**Imprint**



Cover image: www.ingimage.com

This book is a translation from the original published under ISBN 978-613-9-44136-5.

Publisher:
Sciencia Scripts
is a trademark of
Dodo Books Indian Ocean Ltd. and OmniScriptum S.R.L publishing group

120 High Road, East Finchley, London, N2 9ED, United Kingdom
Str. Armeneasca 28/1, office 1, Chisinau MD-2012, Republic of Moldova, Europe
Printed at: see last page
**ISBN: 978-620-8-22939-9**

**Summary:**

Pulpal pathologies constitute the majority of stomatological clinical emergencies and, if treated in a timely manner, they reduce dental mortality. The general objective was to determine the evolution of the treatment of transient serous acute reversible pulpitis (incipient stage) by prolonging the use of eugenol as a pulp sedative up to 96 hours. Methodology: A prospective descriptive observational longitudinal study was carried out in the Stomatological Department of the Manuel "Piti" Fajardo Teaching Polyclinic from March 2022 to February 2023.The population consisted of all patients who attended the stomatological department of the Manuel "Piti" Fajardo University Teaching Polyclinic during the period from March 2022 to February 2023 with acute irreversible serous pulpitis (incipient stage), who after 48 hours of pulp sedation did not achieve a favourable evolution to treatment in the age range of 16 to 35 years and who gave their informed consent to participate in the study.In order to obtain the sample, a purposive sampling by criteria was carried out and it was made up of 32 patients. Results: The study showed that the age group most affected by transient acute serous pulpitis (incipient stage) was 21 to 25 and 26 to 30 years of age, and the sex most affected was female. Conclusions: The evolution of the treatment was considered favourable when, 96 hours after treatment, the symptoms had completely subsided. The majority of patients had a favourable evolution after treatment. Key words: evolution, pulpitis, treatment.

# Table of contents:

## Introduction:

There are several acute pulp pathologies considered reversible, which, if correctly diagnosed and treated, with the use of conservative treatments can prevent tooth loss, the fundamental objective of the stomatologist.[1] Most authors agree that the most frequent cause of pulp lesions is bacterial invasion; microorganisms and their products can reach the pulp either through a solution of continuity in the dentine, caries, accidental exposure, or through the spread of a gingival infection or through the bloodstream. Although the latter route is difficult to prove, some experimental evidence supports this aetiological factor (anacoretic effect).[2]

Robinson and Boling[3] discussed anachoresis pulpitis and explained that bacteria can circulate through the bloodstream and colonise or accumulate at sites of inflammation such as in pulp inflammation, for example, caused by a physical or mechanical irritant and this could be one of the explanations for pulp necrosis after trauma (physical irritant). [2]

Branström and Lind[4] , among others, reported that pulp changes can occur even in the presence of incipient caries represented by demineralisation limited to the enamel, which appears as white spots without an actual cavity, or bacterial invasion through fracture of a tooth exposing the pulp to oral fluids and micro-organisms. [4]

Kakehashi et al. (1965)[5] confirmed the importance of micro-organisms in the aetiology of pulpal pathologies, in which they concluded that without the presence of micro-organisms no pulpal or periapical pathologies develop. [5]

According to Lasala A[6] , there have been two problems for several decades that allow us to agree on the knowledge of pulp pathology, which is important for the planning of a rational therapy. The first of these is the near impossibility of knowing and diagnosing the histopathological lesion. The dentist collects the clinical and radiographic data and then, in a methodical and orderly way, can arrive at an anatomopathological diagnosis, but unfortunately, in most cases there is no correlation between the clinical findings and the histopathological findings, which means a frustration in the desire to know the pulp disorder in detail: "the basic goal for treatment planning".The second problem is of a semantic nature, as the different terminologies and classifications published by researchers, very well reasoned and of great scientific value, have caused controversy and dissent, without ever facilitating their clinical and care application, an objective that should be paramount in the development of a classification or terminology. [6]

Several researchers such as Mitchell and Tarplee, Baume and Fiore-Donno, Pheulpin et al., Seltzer and Bender, Hess, among others cited by Lasala[6,7] agree that purely histopathological classifications are important in scientific research, but for professional practice, to assist in deciding an accurate treatment plan, a clinical or therapeutic classification should be preferred and in this regard there has been considerable controversy, even over the years numerous authors have proposed various classifications of pulpal pathology. [6,7]

Worldwide, the most frequently encountered pulp diagnoses are acute pulpitis, and their behaviour varies between countries because of factors such as the existing health care system, culture, dietary habits, economy and environment.[8]

In Mexico in 2016, Mendiburu et al[9] conducted a study at the Faculty of Dentistry of the Autonomous University of Yucatan, reporting that 63% had pulp disease. [9]

Pulpitis is the second most common disease of the oral cavity and accounts for 40.28% of dental emergencies according to a study by the University of Zulia and the Research Institute of the Faculty of Dentistry of Venezuela 2017.[10]

Nalliah et al.[11] , 2018 conducted a study to determine the prevalence of hospital emergency department visits attributed to pulpal disease in the United States in 2018. They concluded that a total of 403,149 emergency department visits had a primary diagnosis code for pulpal disease. The average age was 32 years. [11]

Flores Cango, 2017[12] , in a study conducted in Ecuador out of 237 cases 32% suffered irreversible pulp pathologies and in another study conducted in the Uayma Health Centre, Yucatan, Mexico[12] out of 100 cases 67% suffered this pathology. [12]

Between January 2017 and July 2018 in Las Tunas, Cuba, a study was conducted in 1764 patients with irreversible pulpitis caused by dental caries. The age groups most affected were 25-34 years, with 41.2 %, and 35-59 years, with 39.6 %.[15]

León[13] , carried out a study on the characterisation of pulp pathologies in a sample of 222 patients in the city of Cienfuegos. A form was used which included the variables of age and sex, tooth groups, with the results showing that the most affected age group and sex predilection was between 35 and 59 years, the most affected tooth groups were the lower molars followed by the upper molars. Of these pathologies, 72.9% were caused by dental caries. [13]

Parejo, García, Montoro, Herrero, Herrero, Mayán[14] , carried out a study in Havana where 162 students were diagnosed with this pathology.

In the municipality of Santo Domingo there is a very high number of patients with acute pulp pathologies which, in some cases due to lack of knowledge and in others due to lack of resources, lead stomatologists to carry out invasive and extraction treatments on teeth that can be treated conservatively. The aim of this study is to reduce dental mortality and, therefore, reduce the number of patients requiring prosthetic treatment.

Despite the fact that this pathology is so common, there is no evidence of previous research on this issue in the municipality.

In view of the above, the following scientific problem will be posed:

What will be the evolution of the treatment of transient serous acute reversible pulpitis (incipient stage) prolonging the use of eugenol as a pulp sedative up to 96 hours in patients attending the stomatological service of the Manuel "Piti" Fajardo University Teaching Polyclinic during the period from March 2022 to February 2023 with this pathology and who after 48 hours of pulp sedation do not achieve a favourable evolution with the treatment?

## Objectives:

General Objective:

To determine the evolution of the treatment of transient serous acute reversible pulpitis (incipient stage) by prolonging the use of eugenol as a pulp sedative up to 96 hours.

Specific Objectives:

1. Describe the sample according to age and sex.
2. Characterise the pathology according to clinical variables of interest.
3. To establish the relationship between the clinical variables of pulp pathology and the evolution of treatment.

# Theoretical framework:

## 1. Pulp

### 1.1 Pulp embryology

The pulp derives from the neural crest, the cells of the cephalic neural crest originate from the ectoderm and migrate along the plate towards the upper and lower jaws contributing to the formation of the dental organs. These dental organs neighbouring the lamina undergo cellular activity thanks to thousands of mesenchymal cells that proliferate at the same time as the dental papilla originates. [16]

The pulp is a mesenchymal connective tissue derived from the dental papilla. It is in the sixth week of gestation, in the ectoderm, that tooth formation begins. Cohen. Each dental follicle begins its process of differentiation into specific tissues starting with the formation of the future enamel around the dental papilla.[16]

Initially, a horseshoe shape will be observed where the future dental organs are deposited, one vestibular and the other lingual, which will later mature to form the two dentitions that we know. [16]

In the tenth week of gestation, its formation can be seen in the cap stage. The dental papilla is surrounded by the two enamel organs and a loose fibrous connective tissue known as the dental sac. [16]

The enamel organ is the precursor of dental enamel and from the dental papilla derives dentine and pulp, which is why the pulp system is known as the dentine-pulp organ or complex as they share the same embryonic origin. [17]

The dental sac is ultimately responsible for the formation of the periodontal ligament, while guiding root formation. [17]

When the dental papilla is forming, a rich network of capillary vessels surrounded by a large number of connective tissue cells and fibres can be observed. [17]

The dental papilla influences the differentiation of ectodermal tissues that form the inner enamel epithelium in the direction of the ameloblasts. Consequently, the cellular activity of the ameloblasts is stimulated by underlying odontoblasts that first form the dentine of the cusps. [17]

When the inner and outer enamel epithelia fuse to form the Hertwing's epithelial sheath invaginating into the underlying connective tissue thus determining the future amelocemental junction. At some point the Hertwing's epithelial sheath will disintegrate into the tooth sac to stimulate connective tissue cells to differentiate into cementoblasts which will then be deposited on the outer surface of the dentine also in creation to initiate the process of root formation. So there will also be a dentine cementum junction. When the epithelial sheath fails to detach from the enamel organs and still invaginates into the connective tissue, enamel pearls form on the root surface. [18]

The first signs of dentine formation coincide with the first maturation of the pulp, which then consists of cells, an extracellular medium of collagen and ground substance. It is at this primary stage of maturation that the first sympathetic vessels and nerves that will become the future vasculonervous bundle are also evident. Shortly thereafter, when the root is in the formative period, sensory nerves develop, which explains why some newly erupted primary or permanent teeth do not have high sensitivity and may vary the response of some endodontic tests.[17]

Once the predentine is formed by the odontoblasts, the dental pulp proper is formed and coincides with the secretion of enamel by the ameloblast. [18]

As the pulp cells proliferate and mature, tooth eruption takes place, stimulating root formation. While the roots are forming the root sheath is held in place allowing root morphology. If it is interrupted by the abrupt presence of a vessel or bundle, a canal different from the original one is formed. However, by genetic coding, the sheath undergoes divisions which will lead to the formation of more roots. [17]

While the odontoblasts form root dentine, the root sheath is interrupted by connective tissue cells of the tooth sac and the cementoblasts that will cover the future root differentiate. The cementum then derives from the tooth sac. If some cells of the root sheath remain in the future periodontal ligament they will be called Mallasez epithelial remnants which will be precursors of periapical inflammatory lesions or form neoplasms or root cysts. [16]

When two or more roots are formed, the root sheath is practically interrupted by a horizontal cervical diaphragm. [16]

Other lateral canals are formed when the epithelial sheath is interrupted by fibres of the periodontal ligament during its insertion. Abrupt disintegration of the epithelial sheath also leads to the formation of accessory canals. [17]

The apical foramen or greater apical foramen is formed by genetic coding when epithelial proliferation ceases and root enlargement stops in relation to the completion of the eruption process. This arrest is preceded by the proliferation of cementoblasts that invaginate into the main dentine canal. [18]

It should be remembered that tooth eruption and apical formation is much earlier in women than in men. When direct or indirect endodontic therapy is performed on incompletely formed pulps, the prognosis will improve thanks to the abundant irrigation and the high cellular activity present in the area. The formation of the pulp and supporting tissues have the same maturation and similar timing. [16,17] . During dental development, multiple genetic alterations can occur that give rise to malformations in the three fundamental organs of the tooth. These alterations range from a decrease or increase in the number of teeth, as well as morphological alterations such as amylogenesis imperfecta, enamel hypoplasias, hypocalcifications, dentine dysplasia, dental invaginations, taurodontism, ectodermal dysplasia, tricho-dento-osseous syndrome, pulpal dysplasias, regional odontodysplasia, hypophosphatasia, familial hereditary hypophosphatemia and congenital porphyria. [17,18] In addition to these alterations are drug interactions that influence the stages of tissue mineralisation due to the great affinity of some drug components with the calcium ion, as in the case of tetracyclines due to the formation of the tetracycline calcium orthophosphate complex that results in a dark discolouration in the form of bands on dental surfaces. The 26th week is when the foetus is most sensitive to these drugs, and between 2 months and 2 years of age the teeth may become pigmented and hypoplastic. [17]

The consumption of endocrine hormones alters root formation so it is suggested to avoid their consumption while the teeth are in this period. Please consult about eruption, root formation and apical formation times according to age and sex. [16]

Radiation is another factor influencing tooth formation but directly dependent on the intensity and duration of exposure to radiotherapy treatment.[17]

## 1.2 Histology of the pulp

The dental pulp is a connective tissue that supports a series of structures vital for its survival. It is composed of a matrix of collagen arranged in the form of interlacing fibres suspended in a protein-rich substance of gelatinous consistency that allows the transport of nutrients resulting in a lax and resilient connective tissue with the ability to distend, but immersed in a non-stretchable cavity called the pulp cavity. [18]

This pulp cavity is located inside the tooth and is well differentiated inside the crown, called the pulp chamber, and inside the roots, called the canal or duct. [18]

The periphery of the dental pulp is the critical zone from the endodontic point of view, since it is the zone richest in cells with the capacity to differentiate, below it a zone poor in cells and more internally the pulp itself rich in fibres behaving as the skeleton of the pulp. This zone rich in cells and located peripherally in intimate contact with the underlying dentine is formed by odontoblasts organised in a palisade attached to the predentine which is a mesh of dentine that has not yet mineralised. [17,18]

A cytoplasmic extension is detached from the peripheral odontoblast, which passes through the predentine and enters the dentinal tubule. This dentinal tubule is surrounded by extratubular dentine and in turn by an intertubular dentine that connects the tubules to each other. There is also a dentine that internally covers the tubules called intratubular dentine. All these types of tubular dentine have distinguishing characteristics. Within the tubule, the odontoblast extension travels surrounded by an intertubular fluid that holds it in suspension and occupies one third of the actual length of the tubule; the remaining two thirds only contain fluid. [17,18]

Odontoblasts are responsible for the formation of pulp and all types of dentine whether embryonic or post-embryonic. [18]

The cellular economy of the pulp involves not only odontoblasts but also fibroblasts, the latter being responsible for the formation of collagen fibres and can also differentiate into other cell types through external stimuli or ageing. Other cell types are also present, such as defence cells of the immune system like macrophages, lymphocytes, leukocytes and polymorphonuclear cells; plasma cells and mast cells will be part of the cellular economy during inflammatory processes. Consequently, odontoblasts can also differentiate into odontoclasts. [18]

In summary, the dentin-pulp complex is represented by the already mineralised dentine, a predentine that is less complex and compact than dentine, an odontoblastic zone or layer rich in this type of cells, a subodontoblastic zone or layer not rich in cells and the pulp itself rich in fibres and vascular elements.[18]

Peripheral pulp zone

- Adjacent to the calcified dentine and next to the predentine, there are odontoblastic cells, within it is a subodontoblastic layer called the Weil cell-free zone (an area of mobilisation and replacement of odontoblasts). [19]

Central pulp area

- The main cells are fibroblasts, the main extracellular components are ground substance and collagen. [19]

Fibroblasts

- They are the main cells of the pulp. They synthesise and secrete most of the extracellular components (collagen and ground substance), and remove excess collagen or participate in its replacement in the pulp by resorption of collagen fibres (through the action of lysosomal enzymes, which digest collagen components). [19]

Odontoblast

- It is the cell responsible for dentinogenesis, located at the periphery of the pulp. Its main function is the production of dentine. They originate from the peripheral mesenchymal cells of the dental papilla. [19]

Defence and other cells

- We find defence cells such as histiocytes, macrophages, polymorphonuclear leukocytes, lymphocytes. Histiocytes and macrophages eliminate bacteria and foreign bodies. Leukocytes are involved in pulp inflammation. Lymphocytes are involved in the formation of lesions and immune reactions. [19]

Structural and extra-structural elements

- Composed of fibres and ground substance. [18]

Fibres

- They form a loose reticular structure to support other structural elements of the pulp.[18]
- The fibres found in the pulp are mainly type I and type III collagen.[18]

Basic substance

- It is an amorphous gel-like mass, consisting mainly of complexes of proteins, carbohydrates, water, lipopolysaccharides and proteins. [18]
- The ground substance surrounds and supports the structures and is the medium through which metabolites and waste products are transported from the cells to the vessels. [18]

Pulp blood supply

- The main function of the microcirculation is the transport of nutrients and waste products to and from the tissues. [19]
- At the apex and extending through the central pulp, one or more arterioles branch into terminal arterioles, which extend into the odontoblastic layer where they form the capillary plexus.[19]
- At the apex, multiple venules emerge from the pulp; these venules communicate with blood vessels draining the periodontal ligament or the adjacent alveolar bone.[19]

## 1.3 Pulp physiology

The pulp plays an important role throughout life because it is responsible for 4 important functions. [20]

Formative

Once the pulp is formed in the mesoderm through the dental papilla, it meets the internal enamel epithelium from the ectoderm, activates the underlying odontoblasts and initiates the process of dentine formation, which forms the crown and later the root or roots. Dentine forms throughout life at different times and with different characteristics. For example, developmental dentine is the first dentine to form. Then an initial dentine, orthodentine or primary dentine is formed; this dentine is tubular and somewhat disorganised because the odontoblasts are not organised. Then we find the mantle dentine, which is the one in intimate contact with the enamel and cementum. As the dentine forms in a central direction, the number of dentinal tubules decreases due to the multiple forces it undergoes. This type of dentine is known as functional, or secondary dentine because it is more stimulus related; it is also known as circumpulpal dentine and corresponds to the largest mass of dentine under the mantle. [20]

If the external stimuli are intense, an atypical dentine is formed as a result of operative, abrasive, acidic, caries, erosive procedures, etc. It is a kind of scar dentine in compensation for the dentine lost by the external stimulus. This type of dentine is tertiary, reparative, irregular or defensive. Langerland[20] has proposed to call it irritational dentine. This dentine does not have much sensitivity as the direction of the tubule and the direction of the odontoblast extension is disrupted. [20] A higher degree of trauma could obliterate the lumen of the dentinal tubules as a form of defence. This dentine is better known as traumatic dentine and its density is such that it appears denser and yellowish. To such a degree tissue aggregation occurs and condenses and traps matrix and cells that it is known as osteodentine. Some authors believe that even fibroblasts contribute to the formation of this dentine, although this is not their function.[20]

Nourishing

The pulp keeps the dentine alive by constantly supplying nutrients and oxygen to the odontoblasts and their extensions. It also provides constant fluid to the dentinal tubules. This nourishing function comes from the subodontoblastic capillary plexus at the periphery of the pulp. The vasculonervous bundle enters through a foramen of 0.1mm diameter to arborise in the widest part of the pulp in the chamber which may be 2-5mm. Forming a bundle of venules, arterioles, lymphatics and sensory nerve endings. [20, 21]

Sensitive

All connective tissue, and the pulp is no exception, requires neurological input to provide this function with two features, vasomotor control and defence. Vasomotor control governs the ability of the blood vessel muscle to dilate or contract, thus regulating blood volume and intrapulp pressure. This allows the central nervous system to recognise an aggressor and initiate a defensive response before an irreversible process is initiated by controlling contractions and vasodilatations through afferent and efferent lines. However, these sensory responses are multi-dependent on the individual and are related to intensity, gender, emotions, motivations, personality, character, past experiences, interpretation of pain, etc. [21]

The afferent neurons of the pulp come from and are directed in relation to the V cranial nerve, the trigeminal nerve, carrying the impulse to the thalamus where it becomes conscious and from there to the cerebral cortex where the response is initiated. Recall that a large part of the nerve fibres of the pulp are type C amyelinic and require, like any nerve fibre, depolarisation to initiate the pain response. Finally, the response reaches a group of nerve fibres located in the cellular area of the pulp known as Raschkow's plexus[21] type A - delta myelinated and the already known C amyelinated. These nerve fibres enter the tubules no more than one third in a coronal direction, which would explain the discrepancy in pain perception in some patients. [21] Defensive

Any response of the pulp to an aggressor results in a painful response, accompanied by vasodilatation and inflammation that recruits cells of the immune system that provide a cellular response system.[21]

## 2. Dolorbucodental

Evoking the term defined by the International Association for the Study of Pain, it could be defined as an unpleasant sensory and emotional experience, related to real or apparent damage to the oral-facial tissues and described as if this damage had occurred. [22]

### 2.1 Common causes of oral pain.

They have different origins, and can be caused by infectious, traumatic, autoimmune, deficiency and not infrequently tumoural lesions. [22]

- Infectious lesions: these are caused by bacteria, viruses or fungi that cause gingivitis, stomatitis, pericoronaritis, alveolitis, pulpitis, periodontitis, dentoalveolar abscesses and ulcerations of various kinds. [22]
- Traumatic injuries: accidental injuries such as trauma, mechanical injuries or those resulting from invasive stomatological interventions, such as exodontia, prostheses or various oral surgeries. [22]

- Autoimmune lesions: these are less common, usually involving the whole body, but have repercussions in the oral cavity such as scleroderma, which causes gingival recession, or dermatomucomyositis, which causes retractile cheilitis and subgingival lesions. [22]
- Deficiency-type lesions: avitaminosis mainly due to vitamin E and B complex deficiency, which predispose to inflammatory lesions and infections. There is another type of non-inflammatory pain related to fluid leaks in the dentinal tubules of various substances, such as hypertonic glucose or cold liquids (dentinal pain).[22]

## 2.2 Classification of oral pain

There are many classifications based on various criteria, including: quality of sensation, site of tissue damage, speed of nerve impulse propagation, among others. The most commonly used classification refers to the location of the receptor (somatic or visceral pain) and the speed of transmission of the pain signal through the nociceptive pathways (fast or slow pain). [23]

The origin of oral pain is related to the affected structure; it can be caused by noxas that produce inflammation (infections, trauma, stomatological manipulations, autoimmune and deficiency disorders) and affect different tissues. [23]

In fact, somatic damage is that which occurs when structures such as gingival and subgingival tissues, the bony structures of the jaws, as well as blood vessels are affected. Nociceptors detect damage to these structures. [23]

On the other hand, neuropathic pain is that which arises from direct injury to nerve structures (nerve trunks and fibres). For example, dentinal pain, caused by the circulation of hypertonic or very cold liquids through the dentinal tubules. Innervating these tubules are A-delta nociceptor nerve fibres, which detect the fluid inside the tubules, thus initiating the pain process. However, inflammatory lesions of the dental pulp also have a neuropathic component, as they involve the sensory fibres found in the pulp; trigeminal neuralgia is also typical and is treated by neurology. [23] There is also the so-called visceral pain, which originates in the capsules of the solid viscera (kidneys, liver) and in the hollow viscera, either because they stretch or contract exaggeratedly (stomach and intestines). Injury to the salivary glands can also cause this type of pain. [23]

## 2.3 Biochemical and physiological mechanisms involved in the origin of the oral pain signal.

In oral pain due to inflammation, a typical positive feedback mechanism is represented; the nociceptive stimulus on the tissue (pulp, periodontal, among others) promotes the release of chemical mediators from 2 origins: from the plasma (bradykinin) and from the injured cells (prostaglandin E2 -PGE2-). Both act on the nerve ending, which is sensitised by the action of PGE2; bradykinin completes its excitation, producing the generation of action potentials in the nociceptive fibre and, therefore, pain. [24]

Thus, the nerve ending is not only excited, but has the capacity to release neuropeptides (substance P and calcitonin genetically related peptide -CGRP-), which act on the mast cells surrounding the blood vessels and these release histamine and cytokines from their granules and prostaglandins from their membranes; they increase vasodilation as well as increase vascular permeability. In addition, they increase the delivery of fresh chemical mediators to the area, promote further nerve fibre activation and perpetuate inflammation. [23] All the events described are important to know that, in a surgical procedure that involves prolonged and traumatic time, the level of chemical mediators will increase in the compromised tissue and, therefore, the inflammatory process will increase, as well as pain; an aspect that should be taken into account in traumatic and prolonged exodontia, or any other endobuccal surgery treatment. [25]

### 2.4 Duration time of oral pain, its intensity and dimensions.

Differentiating oral pain according to its duration is very important, as it contributes to the diagnosis of the underlying disease (biological or warning function of pain) and consequently to the type of treatment to be applied. It is classified, according to its duration, into acute (if it lasts less than 3 months) and chronic (if it lasts more than 3 months). Its intensity has been very difficult to determine, given its strong subjective component (by the patient's reference or by using a scale to measure it). [23]

There are 3 levels of pain intensity:

- Pain of mild intensity: pain that, regardless of its origin, does not compromise the sufferer's daily activities, can be tolerated and treatment is optional; on the analogue pain scale it is pain below 4. [24]
- Moderate intensity: requires immediate treatment, if not relieved it can interfere with the sufferer's daily activities and create a state of moderate anxiety. [24]
- Severe pain: clearly interferes with the patient's activities, prostrates and immobilises, creates a state of extreme anxiety, and therefore requires urgent treatment. [24]

In the stomatological field, the cause of pain of maximum intensity or severe pain is considered to be that produced by surgery for the extraction of third molars, which is not only the most traumatic and painful, but can also be more intense hours after the procedure. Equally severe, but less than that referred to third molars, is considered to be the discomfort produced by the extraction of retained roots. It is accepted that procedures involving bone tissue are the most severe in intensity, unlike soft tissue surgery or simple extractions that produce mostly moderate pain. [24]

Regardless of the duration of the pain or its tissue origin, the intensity often determines the therapeutic approach, i.e. it indicates whether one drug should be used for mild or moderate pain or another for severe pain. It should also be taken into account that the magnitude of the injury is not always proportional to the intensity of the pain, since small injuries can cause severe pain intensity.[24]

## 2.5 Current theories on oral pain perception

The mechanisms that transmit thermal, chemical, electrical or tactile stimuli through dentine are not fully understood. In addition, the fact that dentine is innervated or that odontoblasts are transducers of nerve impulses, as well as the traditional view that dentine irritation is the only stimulant of nociceptors, are controversial. [25]

Several theories of dentine sensitivity have been postulated:

- Dentine nerve stimulation (dentine innervation): The fact that dentine is innervated has been a matter of debate. Also, studies on dental innervation based on chemical staining of nerve elements are somewhat misleading. Traditionally, silver salts have been used to identify the distribution of nerve fibres because nerve tissue has an affinity for it; however, they also stain collagen and reticular fibres. [25]
- Dentin receptor theory: Odontoblasts and their extensions are considered to function as dentin receptor mechanisms and are therefore involved in the initiation and transmission of sensory stimuli in dentin; however, the synaptic junctions, which are essential for nerve conduction between nerve cells and odontoblast extensions, have not been fully identified. [25]
- Hydrodynamic theory: In 1963 Brannstrom[25] hypothesised that dentine pain and odotontoblastic displacement are related. Dentinal pulp fluid expands and contracts in response to the stimulus. The contents of dentinal tubules move into or out of the pulp in response to a given stimulus, because liquids have a higher coefficient of expansion than solid dentine. There is rapid outward movement of pulp dentinal fluid by capillary attraction through exposed dentinal tubule openings. Thus, thermal stimulation, scaling, cavity preparation and sugar placement cause outflow of dentine fluid. [25]

## 3. Pulpal and periapical diseases

### 3.1 Definition.

Pulp disease: This is the response of the pulp in the presence of an irritant, to which it first adapts and as far as necessary opposes, organising itself to resolve favourably the slight injury or dysfunction caused by the aggression, if this is serious (such as pulp injury or very deep caries) the pulp reaction is more violent as it is unable to adapt to the new situation, it tries at least a long and passive resistance towards chronicity; if it does not succeed, rapid necrosis occurs and even if it achieves the chronic state it perishes completely after a certain time. [26]

Periapical disease: Includes inflammatory and degenerative diseases of the tissues surrounding the tooth mainly in the apical region. Pulp disease, if not treated in time or properly, spreads along the canal and reaches the periapical tissues through the foramen. This process can be violent, acute, slow and generally asymptomatic, thus constituting a chronic process. [26]

### 3.2 Epidemiology

The majority of emergencies in our dental clinics are due to pulp and periapical pathologies, because despite prophylactic preventive and curative measures against dental caries, it is still the most widespread disease in humans with an average prevalence of 90 %. Its behaviour varies from country to country, influenced by lifestyle, environment and health care system. [27]

Therefore, dental caries has so far been the most frequent aetiological factor in the incidence of pulp disease, however, dental trauma is increasing considerably and may become the number one aetiological factor in pulp tissue loss in the future.[27]

### 3.3 Classification of Pulpal and Periapical States.

Histopathological classification

Most authors classify pulp diseases as inflammatory or pulpitis, regressive and degenerative or pulposis and pulp death or necrosis.

Pathogenic Classification of Pulpal Inflammation (Baume, Fiore Donno and Pheulpin et al.) [27]

- Acute inflammation (incipient pulpitis): vasodilatation, circulatory stasis, interstitial haemorrhage, oedema, intravascular mobilisation of leukocytes.
- Acute inflammation (acute pulpitis): localised diapedesis of neutrophils and eosinophils, serous exudation, microabscesses, phagocytosis.
- Chronic inflammation (chronic pulpitis): Diffuse infiltration of lymphocytes and plasmacytes, mobilisation of histiocytes and macrophages, calcific and fibrous

degeneration, ulcer formation at the site of exposure. [27]

- Abscess inflammation (suppurative pulpitis): Microabscess, fibrous encapsulation, multiple abscesses with liquefaction necrosis, generalised oedema and serous exudation, thrombosis. [27]
- Acute necrobiosis: total diffuse phlegmonous inflammation, total infection, secondary infection, gangrene. [27]
- Chronic necrobiosis: general plasmacytic infiltration, cystic lysis with liquefaction necrosis, vacuoles. [27]

Histopathological Classification of Pulpal Inflammation (Rebel 1954)28

- Prestatic hyperaemia
- Acute pulpitis
  - Serous pulpitis

Partially circumscribed Fully circumscribed Totally diffuse

  - Purulent pulpitis

  Circumscribed partial abscess totally diffuse

- Chronic pulpitis
  - Closed pulpitis

    Chronic serous Chronic purulent Chronic purulent Internal granulomatosis

  - Open pulpitis

    Ulcerative Granulomatous

  - Infectious necrosis
  - Gangrenous necrosis
  - Apical periodontitis

Anatomical Classification of Pulpal States (Seltzer and Bender 19)29

- Intact pulp without inflammation
- Atrophic pulp (pulposis)
- Acute pulpitis
- intact pulp with chronic inflammatory cells (transitional stage)
- Chronic pulpitis Partial

With partial necrosis due to liquefaction

With partial coagulation necrosis

- Chronic total pulpitis
- Total pulp necrosis

Histopathological Classification of Pulpal Diseases (Grossman 1965)[30]

- Hyperemia
- Pulpitis

Acute serous

Acute suppurative

Chronic ulcerative

Chronic hyperplastic

- Degenerations

Calcium

Fibrous

Atrophic

Grease

Internal resorption

- Pulp necrosis or gangrene[30]

Clinical Classification

The clinical classification of pulp disease is based primarily on symptoms. There is no clinical correlation between histopathological findings and existing symptoms. The value of clinical classification lies in its use in the clinic to determine the proper care and treatment, endodontic prognosis and even the prosthetic needs of the tooth. [30]

Clinical Classification of the Faculty of Dentistry of the Central University of Venezuela based on Baume and Fiore-Donno (1962).[31]

- Class I or Grade I: Asymptomatic Vital Pulp; Pulps that are asymptomatic, injured or accidentally exposed or close to a deep caries or deep cavity, but susceptible to be protected by pulp capping. [31]
- Class II or Grade II: Reversible pulpitis; Pulps with painful clinical symptoms, but amenable to conservative therapy by drugs, pulp capping or vital pulpotomy. [31]
- Class III or Grade III: Irreversible pulpitis; Pulps with clinical symptoms, in which conservative treatment is not indicated, and pulp removal and corresponding canal filling must be carried out. [31]

- Class IV or Grade IV: Necrotic pulp without chronic apical periodontitis; Necrotic pulps with infection of root dentine, requiring antiseptic root canal therapy. [31]
- Class V or Grade V: Necrotic pulps with periapical lesion or chronic apical periodontitis. [31]

<u>Clinical Classification by Pumarola S. and Canalda S. based on Walton and Torabinejad</u>[32]

- Reversible Pulpitis

Symptomatic (Pulpal Hyperemia)

Asymptomatic

- Irreversible Pulpitis

Symptomatic: Serous or Purulent

Asymptomatic: Ulcerative or Hyperplastic

- Pulp necrosis

<u>Grossman's Clinical Classification of Pulpal Diseases (11ª edition)</u>[33]

Pulp inflammation (pulpitis)

- Reversible pulpitis

Symptomatic (acute)

Asymptomatic (chronic)

- Irreversible pulpitis

Acute

- abnormally sensitive to cold
- abnormally heat sensitive

Chronicle

- asymptomatic with pulp exposure
- hyperplastic pulpitis
- internal resorption

- Pulp degeneration

Calcium (radiographic diagnosis)

Other (histopathological diagnosis)

- Necrosis

Grossman's Clinical Classification of Periapical Diseases (1st edition)[33] Acute periradicular diseases.

- Acute alveolar abscess
- Acute apical periodontitis

Vital

Non-vital

- Chronic periradicular diseases with area of rarefaction

Chronic alveolar abscess

Granuloma

Cyst

Osteitis condensans

External root resorption

Clinical Classification of Pulpal and Periapical Conditions [34]

- Initial pulpitis (reversible pulpitis).

Pulpal hyperemia.

Transient pulpitis.

- Acute irreversible pulpitis.

Serous pulpitis.

Suppurative pulpitis

- Irreversible chronic pulpitis.

Ulcerative.

Hyperplastic

- Pathological resorptions of teeth.

External resorptions

Internal resorptions

- Pulp necrosis.

Pulp degeneration

Calcifications.

- Acute periapical processes.

Apical periodontitis

Acute abscess.

- Chronic periapical processes

Chronic abscess

Apical granuloma

Apical cyst.

Clinical Classification of Pulpal and Periapical Conditions[35]

In our country it has now been decided to use a classification based on clinical symptoms and radiographic examination in order to make it simple and practical to diagnose and select the appropriate therapy.

- Asymptomatic vital pulp.
- Dentine hyperaesthesia.
- Reversible inflamed pulp.
- Inflamed pulp degenerating to irreversible.
- Necrotic pulp without area of apical rarefaction.
- Necrotic pulp with area of apical rarefaction.

Classification of pulp and periapical diseases according to Tobón and inserting the histopathological classification described by Álvarez Valls.[35]

- Vital pulp:

Reversible state.

Irreversible state.

- Non-vital pulp:

Chronic condition.

Acute state.

- Reversible vital pulp:

Pulpal hyperemia.

Transient acute serous pulpitis (incipient stage).

- Irreversible vital pulp:

Acute serous pulpitis (installed).

Acute suppurative pulpitis.

Internal resorptions.

Chronic granulomatous and ulcerative pulpitis.

- Chronic non-vital pulp:

Chronic alveolar abscess.

Apical granuloma.

Apical cyst.

Pulp necrosis.

- Acute non-vital pulp:

Apical periodontitis.

Acute alveolar abscess.

**3.4 Diagnosis and treatment of reversible and** irreversible **vital pulp diseases**

Pulpal hyperemia.

Initial reversible pulpitis is present when the microcirculation in the pulp tissue is altered and the velocity of circulating blood increases, when the clinical signs and symptoms correspond to hyperemia, a pre-inflammatory state that denotes blood congestion and constitutes a warning signal indicating that the resistance of the pulp has reached the maximum limit of physiological tolerance, the painful response to mechanical, thermal and electrical stimuli will occur. If at this point, the cause of this condition is not eliminated and pulp irritation continues, it will progress to irreversible pulpitis.[36]

Clinical diagnosis

Questioning: patients and relatives

Refers: Pain

Characteristics of pain:

- Painful sensation to thermal changes (cold and heat).
- Refractory time of the painful sensation is minimal and the sensation disappears quickly when the stimulus ceases.
- No history of spontaneous pain.[37]

Clinical examination:

- Evidence of caries, recurrence or defective filling.
- After-effects of trauma.
- Cracked cusps.
- Cervical lesions with exposed dentine.

- Periodontal disease.
- Occlusal dysfunction.
- Bruxism. [37]

Trans illumination:

- Translucent. [38]

Electrical testing:

- Positive.
- Increased sensitivity. [38]

Thermal testing:

- Positive.
- Sensitive to heat and cold. [38]

Percussion:

- Negative. [38]

Radiographic examination:

- It is only useful for detecting proximal caries if present, as no other radiographic alterations are observed.[38]

Treatment:

Eliminate the cause:

Caries

- Grade II caries: Removal of carious tissue, protection of the dentine-pulp complex and definitive filling. [39]
- Grade III caries: Removal of carious tissue, protection of the dentine-pulp complex and definitive filling. [39]
- Caries grade IV: Removal of carious tissue, protection of the dentine-pulp complex (direct pulp capping with calcium hydroxide) and definitive filling. [39]

Microfiltrations: Remove fillings, assess remaining tissue, place intermediate base and definitive filling. [39]

Trauma: Protection of the dentine-pulp complex and definitive filling. Laser therapy: application of laser in the cavity after removal of carious tissue, filtration filling, or assessment of the traumatised tooth and application in the projection of the root apex.[39]

<u>Transient acute serous pulpitis (incipient stage).</u>

In this phase an inflammatory reaction appears where there is increased blood flow, increased vessel volume, followed by increased vascular permeability, compatible with acute pulpitis, which can be called transient, where by establishing a good diagnosis and adequate protection of the dentin-pulp complex, the pulp can be restored to normal.[40]

Clinical diagnosis

Mild to moderate transient pain that may appear spontaneous, painful sensation to thermal changes and other stimuli that takes longer than in hyperemia to disappear, pain is relieved with analgesics. [40]

Clinical examination:

- Caries, defective fillings and recurrences are observed: Bacterial infection to the pulp is possible when present. [40]
- Bruxism: It is responsible for lesions corresponding to reversible pulpitis. Excessive forces when grinding the teeth cause pulp alterations. [40]
- Periodontal disease: Pulp infection often occurs when we have periodontal disease due to accessory canals leading from the periodontium to the pulp and vice versa. [40]
- Occlusal dysfunction: Physiological changes occur in the pulp tissue due to occlusal disharmonies that create extreme forces in specific areas of the dental arch.[41]
- After-effects of dental trauma: The impact of trauma brings alterations related to reversible pulpitis. If there is a fracture, this is a route of bacterial infection through the exposed dentinal tubules. [41]

Operative treatments performed: Some operative procedures have a traumatic action on the pulp tissue, e.g. cavity preparation without proper cooling, or damage to neighbouring teeth during tooth extraction. [42]

Abrasion or attrition: This condition affects the pulp tissue.

- Electrical test: hypersensitivity.
- Thermal test: hypersensitivity to cold.
- Percussion: negative
- Radiographic examination: only proximal caries could be detected.[41]

Treatment:

It consists first of eliminating the cause of the problem, partial sedation and protection of the dentin-pulp complex by temporary sealing with zinc oxide and eugenol and subsequent definitive obturation. In addition, laser therapy, homeopathy, acupressure, auriculopuncture, suggestion and hypnosis are applied. [43]

Pulpotomy.

If the painful symptomatology does not subside with the previous therapies, a pulpectomy or pulpotomy is performed with the aim of maintaining the pulp of the vital root canals, by means of coronal amputation and the application of a medicine that disinfects and fixes the pulp remnant without devitalising the tissue. This technique consists of removing the entire coronal pulp and leaving the vital tissue of the root canals intact. The stumps of the amputated root pulp are covered with a medication that will promote healing or fixation of the tissue beyond the interface between the medication dressing and the pulp stump.[44]

Before deciding on the application of this therapy, the clinical signs and age of the patient must be assessed and the following requirements must be met:

- Normal bleeding (Not to exceed 5 min).
- Characteristics of the remaining pulp tissue (no liquefaction).
- Degree of coronary destruction, with the possibility of restoration.
- Assessment of the medicine to be used according to age. [44]

Indications:

- Permanent molars with signs of pulp vitality.
- In immature permanent teeth.[45]

Operative technique for performing Pulpotomy:

- Previous periapical X-ray and diagnosis.
- Anaesthesia of the tooth to be treated, never intrapulp.
- Eliminate remaining caries.
- Absolute isolation.
- Cameral access.
- Amputation and removal of chamber pulp with #5 round bur or discoid (sharp spoon).
- Washing with saline or distilled water.
- Haemostasis with sterile cotton wool.
- Laser therapy.
- Avoid detritus and excessive pressure on the remaining pulp tissue.
- Selection of the medicine to be used for pulp protection:

  Calcium hydroxide (young permanent molars and traumatised incisors with immature apices).

Formocresol diluted to one-fifth for 5 minutes (adult permanent molars).

Others such as 2 % glutaraldehyde, ferric sulphate.

- Verification X-ray.
- Laying of intermediate base and restoration.
- Clinical and radiographic controls every 3 months up to one year.[46]

Acute serous pulpitis (installed).

In the initial phase of acute serous pulpitis, changes continue to appear in the blood microcirculatory environment if the disease is not treated in time and as a consequence of the transfer of plasma fluids, there is an increase in blood viscosity and a decrease in the velocity of the circulatory current, establishing the dynamics of inflammation and turning the clinical picture into irreversible pulpitis.[47]

- Clinical diagnosis: the painful symptomatology worsens in relation to the incipient phase.
- Clinical examination: evidence of caries, recurrence, defective filling, dental trauma, conservative treatment, abrasion, attrition, periodontal disease, occlusal dysfunction and bruxism.
- Electrical test: hypersensitivity.
- Thermal test: hypersensitive to cold.
- Percussion: negative.
- Radiographic examination: only proximal caries would be detected.
- Treatment: once the irreversibility of the pulp has been established and defined, pulpotomy or pulporadicular treatment is carried out. Laser therapy, acupuncture and homeopathy techniques are also applied.[48]

Acute suppurative pulpitis

Acute serous pulpitis already in place can rapidly progress to acute purulent pulpitis depending on the resistance and defence of the pulp organ, as well as the degree of bacterial virulence or irritation of the pathogen.[49]

- Clinical diagnosis: pain is spontaneous, moderate to severe, throbbing, constant, persistent, radiating in early stages and localised in advanced stages, increases with postural changes, increases with heat and decreases with cold. [50]
- Clinical examination: evidence of caries, recurrence, defective filling, dental trauma, conservative treatment, abrasion, attrition, periodontal disease, occlusal dysfunction and bruxism.

- Electrical test: positive, increased or decreased sensitivity depending on pulp damage.[51]
- Thermal test: greater sensitivity to heat than to cold.
- Percussion: negative, may be positive in more advanced periods of the condition.
- Radiographic examination: only proximal caries or recurrence of caries would be detected.
- Treatment: pulporradicular in one session. Pulpotomy when pulporradicular treatment is not possible as an alternative treatment. Laser therapy, acupuncture and homeopathy techniques are also applied.[52]

**Chronic granulomatous and ulcerative pulpitis**

Acute pulpitis can slowly evolve into chronic pulpitis through a modification of the relationship between the damaging agent and the host, where the damaging agent does not die, but is only weakened and the acute exudative reaction causes a transition to chronic inflammation and leads to chronic hyperplastic or granulomatous pulpitis, pulp polyp or chronic ulcerated pulpitis. This pulp alteration is usually observed in young patients, as a result of a low intensity and long lasting irritation on a pulp able to resist this irritant action.[53]

- Thermal test: discrete increase to thermal changes.
- Percussion: negative.
- Radiographic examination: extensive carious lesion or coronary fracture communicating with the pulp chamber.
- Treatment: pulporadicular or biopulpectomy. Pulpotomy with calcium hydroxide in teeth with incomplete root formation.[54]

**Internal root resorptions**

Resorption is a condition associated with a physiological or pathological process that results in a loss of tissue substance, such as dentine, cementum and alveolar bone. Internal resorption begins in the pulp cavity. When resorption originates in the crown of the tooth and reaches the enamel, it is called internal resorption.

a pink spot can be seen which is known as a "pink tooth". There is external resorption that starts in the periodontium and affects the outer surface of the tooth and there is idiopathic resorption caused by no apparent cause. This section describes internal resorption, which has always been a mystery that is difficult to decipher.[52]

- Clinical diagnosis: asymptomatic, pain may occur in case of perforation. [53]
- Clinical examination: caries, deep fillings, pulp exposure, sequelae of dental trauma,

pinkish stain at the level of the pulp chamber. [53]

- Electrical test: decreased sensitivity. [53]
- Thermal test: decreased sensitivity. [53]
- Percussion: negative[53]
- Radiographic examination: radiolucent image of enlargement in the pulp chamber or root canal in an asymmetrical shape.[53]
- Treatment: Pulporradicular and sometimes periapical surgery is required. During biomechanical preparation, abundant irrigation should be carried out with 5% sodium hypochlorite, which has great bactericidal power, and a medicinal cure of chemically pure calcium hydroxide associated with camphorated paramonochlorophenol should be applied, thus halting the resorption process and subsequently obturating the root canal, preferably with thermoplastic gutta-percha. Good results have been obtained using laser therapy and homeopathic treatments. [53]

## 4. **Eugenol.**

Eugenol is a phenolic derivative commonly known as clove essence, which can also be extracted from pepper, bay leaves, cinnamon, camphor and other oils. It is oily liquid in consistency, light yellow in colour, with a characteristic aroma, poorly soluble in needle and soluble in alcohol. Clove oil has been used since the 16th century, until Chisolm[55] in 1873, introduced it into dentistry and recommended that it be mixed with zinc oxide to form a zinc eugenolate putty that could be applied directly to carious cavities. As knowledge of its pharmacological properties evolved, its use became more common, specific and selective until today, when it is used in different areas of dentistry for various purposes, mainly for the suppression of pain. Eugenol is used in stomatology, often mixed with zinc oxide, as a temporary filling material, and is a component of oral hygiene preparations. It is sometimes used as a flavouring. It has also been used as a pulp sedative, temporary cementing agent, surgical dressing, root canal filler, topical anaesthetic, tooth protector, disinfectant in root canal fillings and pulp capping.[55]

### **4.1 Pharmacological properties.**

### **Release and diffusion of Eugenol**

When Eugenol binds to zinc oxide, a chelation reaction occurs, forming zinc eugenolate (ZOE). When examined ultrastructurally, ZOE cement consists of zinc oxide grains embedded in a zinc eugenolate matrix, the units of which are bound by Van der Waals forces and interparticle interaction, making the cement mechanically weak. When exposed to an aqueous medium such as saliva or dentinal fluid, hydrolysis of zinc eugenolate occurs, yielding eugenol and zinc hydroxide. Thus the Eugenol released from ZOE can diffuse through the dentine and into the saliva. The release of Eugenol is not markedly affected by the ratio of the zinc oxide-eugenol mixture, but by the thickness of the remaining dentine between the pulp chamber and the ZOE-filled cavity. The ability of Eugenol to diffuse through dentine is affected by several factors such as: the calcium in the dentinal tubules, which forms a chelate with Eugenol, and the binding of Eugenol to the organic matrix of dentine, especially to collagen. [56]

Modes of action

Its effects and postulated mechanisms of action are manifold.

One of the properties attributed to Eugenol is pain relief when applied to dental organs. Eugenol is an irreversible nerve conduction blocker and at low concentrations, it is capable of reducing synaptic transmission in the neuromuscular area. Several studies have concluded that Eugenol inhibits cyclooxygenase, favouring the analgesic and anaesthetic effect by inhibiting prostaglandin biosynthesis. At low concentrations Eugenol reversibly inhibits nerve activity, like a local anaesthetic. After exposure to high concentrations of Eugenol, nerve conduction is irreversibly blocked, indicating a neurotoxic effect. Eugenol also reduces synaptic transmission at the neuromuscular junction. Sensory nerve fibres and their functions play an important role in the generation of the inflammatory response, as sensory nerves in the dental pulp contain vasoactive peptides, such as substance P, calcitonin gene-related peptide, and others. The fact that Eugenol inhibits nerve activity and vascular components of the inflammatory response, as well as the relationship between these elements, may be linked to its possible anti-inflammatory effects.[56]

Eugenol inhibits neutrophil chemotaxis and superoxide anion generation at low (non-toxic) concentrations. Eugenol has been found to act as a competitive inhibitor of prostaglandin H (PGH) synthetase, and prevents the binding of arachidonic acid to this enzyme with the consequent formation of PGH. Clove oil has been shown to be a potent inhibitor of thromboxane formation and platelet aggregation in human blood in vitro. Both prostaglandins (PGs) and leukotrienes (LTs) are important mediators of the inflammatory response. PGE2 and some LTs increase blood flow and vascular permeability, and at physiological concentrations sensitise nerve endings. [56, 57]

The effects of reactive oxygen species are molecular events related to tissue damage. Numerous studies have demonstrated the antioxidant capacity of Eugenol and related compounds (such as isoeugenol) to inhibit lipid peroxidation induced by reactive oxygen species. It also inhibits the formation of superoxide radicals in the xanthine-xanthine oxidase system, as well as the generation of hydroxyl radicals, preventing the oxidation of $Fe^{2+}$ in the Fenton reaction, which generates this radical, one of the most aggressive to tissues, due to all the reactions it triggers. This chemopreventive property may be due to its free radical scavenger activity.[56]

At high concentrations it has a bactericidal effect, an action that has been attributed to phenols by degeneration of proteins, resulting in damage to the cell membrane, whereas at low concentrations it tends to stabilise cell membranes, which prevents the penetration of bacteria into the dentine ducts. The results suggest that Eugenol inhibits the growth of several pathogenic fungal organisms, either alone or in combination (Eugenol - Thymol, Eugenol - Carvacrol), which may be effective in the treatment of oral infectious diseases. The antibacterial effects of zinc oxide - Eugenol and other materials have also been studied against aerobic and anaerobic bacteria.[56, 57]

As we have seen, the pharmacological effects of Eugenol are complex and depend on the concentration of free Eugenol to which the tissue is exposed.[57]

Low concentrations can be obtained by diffusion of the Eugenol from ZOE through the intact dentine layer. The application of obturator ZOE after deep caries excavation could exert sedative anti-inflammatory effects. When applying Eugenol or ZOE in direct contact with vital tissue, high concentrations capable of producing cytotoxic effects on it are released, so it is recommended that direct application of Eugenol should be carried out when the endodontic procedure is for a few days. [57]

The pharmacological actions of Eugenol can negatively affect other important functions of some damaged tissue cells, which is closely related to the way it is used. Thus, Eugenol can inhibit the activity of the periapical nerve, but at the same time high concentrations of Eugenol can also be toxic to the periapical nerve, and both effects can influence the decrease in pain perception. Likewise, through inhibition of the synthesis of prostaglandins and leukotrienes, Eugenol helps in the resolution of inflammation of the periapical tissue, but at the same time, the contribution of prostaglandins, especially PGE2, is of great relevance for this disease, especially PGE2, in bone resorption, as fibroblasts in apical cysts are thought to synthesise PGE2 under lymphocyte stimulation, which stimulates osteoclasts to bone resorption. Eugenol's effect on neutrophil chemotaxis and free radical scavenging may also aid the resolution of apical inflammation through its bactericidal effect, but these inflammatory components also cause tissue damage when the response is exacerbated. [57]

Toxicity

Although its application is common, Eugenol can cause caustic lesions or superficial burns when applied directly and in high concentrations to soft tissues. The severity of damage is proportional to exposure time, dose and concentration. Eugenol has been shown to exhibit both in vivo and in vitro different types of toxicity, such as direct tissue damage, dermatitis, allergic reactions, liver damage, disseminated intravascular coagulation, severe hypoglycaemia, and even death from multiple organ failure. Pure

Eugenol at concentrations greater than 10-4 mol/L has been shown to inhibit cell migration and modify prostaglandin synthesis, affecting cellular respiration, mitochondrial activity and producing severe changes in cell membrane enzyme activity.Other studies have delved into the effects of topical application of clove oil on the labial mucosa, and observed progressive denaturation and fixation of cytoplasm on the surface of the epithelium, followed by tissue liquefaction, oedema, loss of intercellular bridges and dissolution of some superficial muscle fibres. A group of researchers led by Garza Padilla and Toranzo Fernandez, conducted a toxicity study of several Eugenol formulations in rabbits, analysing skin, liver, kidney and brain samples, and obtained as a result severe local toxicity at the site of application, in all cases, practically with similar changes, with a predominance of ischaemic necrosis, probably as a consequence of direct damage and vascular spasms. At high concentrations, Eugenol stimulates the release of superoxide from neutrophils, which increases tissue damage at the site of inflammation.[58]

Eugenol is bactericidal at relatively high concentrations (10-2 to 10-3 mol/L). Brief exposure to 10-2 mol/L Eugenol kills mammalian cells, as does prolonged exposure to 10-3 mol/L. 1 Data from Hume15 have shown that concentrations of Eugenol diffusing through dentine are non-cytotoxic, although low concentrations can also inhibit respiration and cell division. 58

Several biochemical mechanisms have been proposed to explain the cytotoxicity of Eugenol, such as:

- Eugenol can be oxidised by the enzyme peroxidase to a toxic product in rat hepatocytes. [58]
- Eugenol and related compounds were shown to have a high affinity for the plasma membrane due to their lipid solubility. [58]
- Cotmore[58] et al. reported that Eugenol can uncouple oxidative phosphorylation in mitochondria. [58]

These toxic effects of Eugenol may explain why its direct application in cotton pellets on pulp tissue causes exacerbation of pulpitis symptoms. Direct contact between vital tissue and eugenol-containing material can cause tissue damage.[58]

Methodological design:

A prospective descriptive observational longitudinal study was carried out. The research took place in the Stomatological Department of the Manuel "Piti" Fajardo Teaching Polyclinic from March 2022 to February 2023.The population consisted of all patients who attended the stomatological department of the Manuel "Piti" Fajardo University Teaching Polyclinic from March 2022 to February 2023 with acute irreversible serous pulpitis (incipient stage) and who after 48 hours of pulp sedation did not achieve a favourable evolution with treatment, aged between 16 and 35 years, and who gave their informed consent (Appendix 1) to participate in the study.The sample was obtained by purposive sampling by criteria and consisted of 32 patients.

Exclusion criteria:

- Patients with pulp exposure.
- Pregnant patients due to the impossibility of taking X-rays Methodology and methods

Methods:

Empirical: Based on daily practice, experience and observation of the facts, it allowed the final report to be drawn up. The questionnaire is aimed at determining the exact symptoms and characteristics of the pathology in each patient. (Annex 3) Statistical: This method was used for data processing.

Methodology:

The research was carried out in three stages:

Stage I: After a thorough interrogation and detailed clinical examination we arrived at the diagnosis of acute serous transient reversible pulpitis (incipient stage). These data were recorded in the form for each patient (Appendix 2). The patients who presented this pathology and who after 48 hours of pulp sedation did not achieve a favourable evolution to the treatment in the age range of 16 to 35 years and who gave their informed consent, formed the sample of the investigation. The patients were examined by the author in the dental chair, using artificial light and a classification set, at the time of the visit.

Stage II: Management and treatment of transient serous acute reversible pulpitis (incipient stage).

At this point, a cotton swab soaked in eugenol was applied until 96 hours had elapsed. Subsequently, the remission of the symptoms was evaluated a second time and, if this was achieved, we proceeded to the definitive restoration. Of course, we must do our periodic clinical and radiographic check-ups every 3 months. If the pulp is not brought to a normal stage within this time, then a more invasive treatment will be performed.

The percentage method was used for the analysis.

Stage III: Evaluation of the evolution of the treatment.

Treatment was assessed as favourable when the patient's painful symptoms subsided after 96 hours.

The treatment was ineffective when after 96 hours, i.e. after two seal changes, the patient continued to have pain.

Operationalisation of variables

Age: according to age at the time of the study.

- 16-20 years.
- 21-25 years.
- 26-30 years.
- 31-35 years.

Sex: according to biological gender.

- Male.
- Female.

Pain intensity:according to the Melsak scale[59]

- Mild when the Melsak scale is 2.
- Moderate when on the Melsak scale it is 3 and 4.
- Intense when on the Melsak scale it is 5 and 6.

Melsak scale 1-6.

- No pain present.
- Tolerable mild pain.
- Moderate pain.
- Severe pain, but can continue activity.
- Intense pain that makes it difficult to concentrate.
- Intolerable pain.

Nature of pain.

- Provoked (when the pain is provoked by any stimulus)
- Spontaneous (When the pain occurs spontaneously).

Form of presentation of pain.

- Constant (Permanent pain.)
- Intermittent (painful episodes with periods of remission).

Depth of the lesion: distance from the lesion to the pulp chamber. The distance from the pulp chamber to the floor of the cavity after shaping shall be measured by means of a periapical radiograph with a caliper.

- 0.5 mm
- 1.0 mm
- 1.5 mm
- 2.0 mm

Evolution of treatment.

- Favourable (When the painful symptomatology completely disappears 96 hours after treatment).
- Unfavourable (When the painful symptomatology does not subside with the application of the treatment).

Data collection techniques:

- Observation: As a technique, it allowed us to obtain data directly from the patient and the pathology that afflicts him/her.
- Direct questioning: This was carried out by means of patient interviews.
- Forms: (Annex 2) in this case it is fundamental as it provided us with particular data on each patient that allowed us to make an accurate diagnosis and develop an adequate treatment plan.

Processing methods, data analysis and techniques to be used:

The data were stored in a data file with the professional statistical software SPSS version 22 on Windows, the information was presented in statistical tables and graphs, in their description, absolute frequencies, percentages, and percentages were calculated and non-parametric tests such as Chi-square for independence of factors were used for the analysis.

Ethical considerations:

The study was carried out taking into account international ethical standards for experimental and biomedical research with humans (Nuremberg Code, Declaration of Helsinki I and II, United Nations Principles of Medical Ethics, CIOMS Ethical Standards, Universal Declaration on the Human Genome and Human Rights) and national ethical standards such as the principles of Medical Ethics, Ethical Standards of Good Practice in Human Experimentation. These ethical standards were taken into account from the design of the research project, ensuring strict compliance throughout the study process and culminating in the presentation of the results.

The information obtained was used only for this purpose, it was explained to each patient what the study would consist of, making it clear that it would not involve any harm to their health. In this respect, we prepared a model of informed consent that was signed by each patient within the basic principles to be taken into account, in order to satisfy the moral, ethical and legal requirements in research with human beings and not to violate the bioethical principles of beneficence, non-maleficence, autonomy and justice.

Results:

**Table 1.** Distribution according to age and sex in patients with transient acute serous pulpitis (incipient stage). Manuel Piti Fajardo Polyclinic. Santo Domingo (March 2022 to February 2023)

| Age | Sex | | | | Total | |
|---|---|---|---|---|---|---|
| | Female | | Male | | | |
| | No. | % | No. | % | No. | % |
| 16 - 20 | 5 | 15,6 | 3 | 9,4 | 8 | 25,0 |
| 21 - 25 | 5 | 15,6 | 4 | 12,5 | 9 | 28,1 |
| 26 - 30 | 4 | 12,5 | 5 | 15,6 | 9 | 28,1 |
| 31 - 35 | 3 | 9,4 | 3 | 9,4 | 6 | 18,8 |
| Total | 17 | 53,1 | 15 | 46,9 | 32 | 100 |

Source: form

$X^2 = 0.600$ P= 0.897 NOT SIGNIFICANT

A predominance of the female sex was observed with 17 patients, for 53.1% of the total. The male sex was represented by 15 patients, 46.9% of the total, with no significant difference between the two groups.

In terms of age groups, the most represented were 21-25 and 26-30 with 9 patients in each group for a total of 28.1% in each case. In the 21-25 age group, the most represented sex was female with 5 patients and in the 26-30 age group, male. The least represented group was 31-35 with 3 patients in each sex.

There is no dependency relationship between age and sex.

**Table 2.** Pain intensity

| Intensity of pain | No. | % |
|---|---|---|
| Slight | 16 | 50,0 |
| Moderate | 10 | 31,3 |
| Intense | 6 | 18,8 |
| Total | 32 | 100,0 |

Source: form

Pain intensity was measured by the Melsak scale. With scale 2, which was classified as mild there were 16 patients, representing 50.0% of the sample. With scale 3 and 4, classified as mild, there were 10 patients, representing 31.3%. With scale 5 and 6, which were classified as severe, 6 patients were found, representing 18.8% of the total. Mild pain predominated, and severe pain was the least representative.

**Table 3.** Nature of pain.

| Nature of pain | No. | % |
|---|---|---|
| Spontaneous | 9 | 28,1 |
| Provoked | 23 | 71,9 |
| Total | 32 | 100,0 |

Source: form

The nature of the pain was measured as spontaneous or provoked. With spontaneous pain, 9 patients were observed, representing 28.1% of the total. In most of these cases the patients presented spontaneous pain, but not intense and constant. With provoked pain, 23 patients were observed, representing 71.9% of the total, so that the sample was dominated by patients with pain provoked by the stimulus.

**Table 4.** Form of presentation of pain.

| Form of presentation of pain | No. | % |
|---|---|---|
| Flashing | 27 | 84,4 |
| Constant | 5 | 15,6 |
| Total | 32 | 100,0 |

Source: form

The form of pain presentation was measured as intermittent or constant. With intermittent pain, 27 patients were observed, representing 84.4% of the total. With constant pain, 5 patients were observed, representing 15.6% of the total, so that patients with intermittent pain predominated in the sample.

**Table 5.** Depth of the lesion.

| Depth of injury | No. | % |
|---|---|---|
| 2.0 mm | 12 | 37,5 |
| 1.5 mm | 9 | 28,1 |
| 1.0 mm | 7 | 21,9 |
| 0,5 mm | 4 | 12,5 |
| Total | 32 | 62,5 |

Source: form

The distance of the lesion to the pulp chamber was measured with a caliper foot using a periapical radiograph. There were 12 patients where the distance from the lesion to the pulp chamber was 2.0mm representing 37.5%. There were 9 patients in whom the distance was 1.5mm, representing 28.1%. With a depth of 1.0mm there were 7 patients for 21.9%. With a depth of 0.5 mm there were 4 patients representing 12.5%. The closer the lesion was found to the pulp, the worse the prognosis.

**Table 6.** Evolution of treatment

| Evolution of treatment | No. | % |
|---|---|---|
| Favourable | 25 | 78,1 |
| Not favourable | 7 | 21,9 |
| Total | 32 | 100,0 |

Source: form

The evolution of the treatment was considered favourable when, 96 hours after treatment, the symptoms had completely subsided. Of the total number of patients, 25 had a favourable treatment course, representing 78.1% of the total. The evolution of the treatment was not considered favourable when after having prolonged the treatment up to 96 hours, remission of the painful symptoms was not achieved; this occurred in 7 patients, representing 21.9% of the total sample.

**Table 7.** Evolution of treatment according to age.

| Age | Evolution of treatment | | | | Total | |
|---|---|---|---|---|---|---|
| | Favourable | | Not favourable | | | |
| | No. | % | No. | % | No. | % |
| 16 - 20 | 8 | 25,0 | 0 | 0,0 | 8 | 25,0 |
| 21 - 25 | 9 | 28,1 | 0 | 0,0 | 9 | 28,1 |
| 26 - 30 | 6 | 18,8 | 3 | 9,4 | 9 | 28,1 |
| 31 - 35 | 2 | 6,3 | 4 | 12,5 | 6 | 18,8 |
| Total | 25 | 78,1 | 7 | 21,9 | 32 | 100 |

Source: form

X2 = 12,495 P= 0,003 HIGHLY SIGNIFICANT

Treatment was favourable in 25 patients. The age groups with the best response were 16-20 and 21-25 years with 8 and 9 patients respectively. The highest representation was in the 21-25 age group, representing 28.1%. In the 26-30 years age group there were 6 patients and in the 31-35 years age group there were fewer patients who responded favourably to treatment, only 2, representing 6.3%. Therefore, the age group with the highest proportion of patients who did not respond favourably to treatment was precisely

31-35 years of age.

This behaviour showed that the younger the patients, the better their response to treatment.

There is a highly significant dependency relationship between age and treatment outcome.

**Table 8.** Evolution of treatment according to pain intensity.

| Intensity of pain | Evolution of treatment | | | | Total | |
|---|---|---|---|---|---|---|
| | Favourable | | Not favourable | | | |
| | No. | % | No. | % | No. | % |
| Slight | 16 | 50,0 | 0 | 0,0 | 16 | 50,0 |
| Moderate | 7 | 21,9 | 3 | 9,4 | 10 | 31,3 |
| Severo | 2 | 6,3 | 4 | 12,5 | 6 | 18,8 |
| Total | 25 | 78,1 | 7 | 21,9 | 32 | 100 |

Source: form

X2 = 11,910 P= 0,003 HIGHLY SIGNIFICANT

All patients with mild pain responded favourably to treatment, representing 50% of the total. Of the patients with moderate pain, 7 had a favourable response to treatment (21.9%) and 3 had an unfavourable response (12.5%). The majority of patients with severe pain did not respond favourably, 4 did not respond favourably and 2 responded favourably (12.5% and 6.3% respectively).

This behaviour showed that when patients had mild and moderate pain they responded favourably to treatment.

There is a highly significant dependency relationship between pain intensity and treatment outcome.

**Table 9.** Evolution of treatment according to the nature of the pain.

| Nature of pain | Evolution of treatment | | | | Total | |
|---|---|---|---|---|---|---|
| | Favourable | | Not favourable | | | |
| | No. | % | No. | % | No. | % |
| Spontaneous | 6 | 18,8 | 3 | 9,4 | 9 | 28,1 |
| Provoked | 19 | 59,4 | 4 | 12,5 | 23 | 71,9 |
| Total | 25 | 78,1 | 7 | 21,9 | 32 | 100 |

Source: form

$X^2 = 0,962$ P= 0,327 NOT SIGNIFICANT

Patients with provoked pain responded more favourably to treatment than those with spontaneous pain. Of the 23 patients with provoked pain, 19 had a favourable evolution, representing 59.4%. Of the patients with spontaneous pain, 6 out of 9 patients responded favourably to treatment (18.8%) and 3 responded unfavourably (9.4%). Although most of the patients who presented with spontaneous pain also responded well to treatment, there was greater relevance in those who presented with provoked pain.

There is no dependency relationship between the nature of the pain and the evolution of the treatment.

**Table 10.** Evolution of treatment according to the form of presentation of the pain.

| Form of presentation of pain | Evolution of treatment | | | | Total | |
|---|---|---|---|---|---|---|
| | Favourable | | Not favourable | | | |
| | No. | % | No. | % | No. | % |
| Flashing | 24 | 75,0 | 3 | 9,4 | 27 | 84,4 |
| Constant | 1 | 3,1 | 4 | 12,5 | 5 | 15,6 |
| Total | 25 | 78,1 | 7 | 21,9 | 32 | 100 |

Source: form

X2 = 11.715 P= 0.001 HIGHLY SIGNIFICANT

Patients with intermittent pain responded better to treatment than those with constant pain. Of the 27 patients with intermittent pain, 24 had a favourable evolution, representing 75.0% of patients. Of the patients with constant pain, 4 out of 5 patients responded unfavourably to treatment (12.5%) and 1 responded favourably (3.1%).

This behaviour showed that when patients' pain was intermittent, they responded favourably to treatment.

There is a highly significant dependency relationship between the form of pain presentation and treatment outcome.

There is a highly significant dependency relationship between the form of pain presentation and treatment outcome.

**Table 11.** Evolution of treatment according to the depth of the lesion.

| Depth of injury | Evolution of treatment | | | | Total | |
|---|---|---|---|---|---|---|
| | Favourable | | Not favourable | | | |
| | No. | % | No. | % | No. | % |
| 2.0 mm | 12 | 37,5 | 0 | 0,0 | 12 | 37,5 |
| 1.5 mm | 9 | 28,1 | 0 | 0,0 | 9 | 28,1 |
| 1.0 mm | 3 | 9,4 | 4 | 12,5 | 7 | 21,9 |
| 0,5 mm | 1 | 3,1 | 3 | 9,4 | 4 | 12,5 |
| Total | 25 | 78,1 | 7 | 21,9 | 32 | 100 |

Source: form.

X2 = 13.633 P= 0.003 HIGHLY SIGNIFICANT

Patients whose lesion-to-pulp chamber distance measured between 2.0mm and 1.5mm responded favourably to treatment with 12 and 9 patients respectively. The majority of patients who responded unfavourably when the distance between the chamber and the lesion was between 1.0mm and 0.5mm, mostly the latter, representing 9.4%, responded unfavourably.

This behaviour showed that the closer the lesion was to the pulp chamber, the worse the treatment progressed.

There is a highly significant dependency relationship between the depth of the lesion and the evolution of the treatment.

Discussion of the results:

The study found that the age group most affected by transient acute serous pulpitis (incipient stage) was 21 to 25 and 26 to 30 years of age, and the sex was female. These results coincide with those obtained by Jiménez[60] in this age group; however, they differ from the results of Ruiz[61] and Gaviria et al[62] in both sex and age group.Portal Macías[63] reports greater affectation in the 35-49 age group, which is not similar to the present study. In none of the studies is there a statistically significant relationship between age and sex. It is also similar to that of Fernández Cortina[64] , in whose study the female sex predominates.

The peculiarity of pulp pathologies lies in the fact that biological age does not always coincide with pulp age. According to the author's criteria, in the range of 31 to 35 years, the exposure time of the tooth to different harmful stimuli has been longer, and the regeneration capacity of the pulp tissue is lower. She also argues that, at this stage, in general, there is greater responsibility for work and social activities, prioritising these, and not worrying about their oral health.

Quiñonez[65] argues that the greater gender impact could be linked to the fact that women are more interested in receiving dental treatment to improve their aesthetics and functionality, or that women may be more susceptible to dental morbidity.

Boltacz and Laszkiewics[66,] report different results, with the conditions occurring more frequently in men.

Pain intensity was measured by the Melsak scale. Mild pain was predominant, and severe pain was the least representative. Patients with mild pain all responded favourably to treatment. Patients with severe pain mostly did not respond favourably. This behaviour shows that when patients had mild and moderate pain they responded favourably to treatment. According to Perez et al[68] , intensity is related to the emotional reaction to the stimuli that trigger it, pain perception, pain threshold and tolerance capacity, which vary between individuals. It is influenced by cognitive, emotional and motivational factors and is related to socio-cultural factors. The occurrence of pain in reversible processes is provoked, and in irreversible processes it is spontaneous.

According to the nature of the pain in the sample, there was a predominance of patients with provoked pain to the stimulus. Patients with provoked pain responded more favourably to treatment than those with spontaneous pain. This behaviour demonstrates that when the pain presented by the patients was provoked to the stimulus, they responded favourably to the treatment.

González and Montero[63] report that, depending on its quality, pain can be sharp or continuous, which depends on the functional properties of the trigeminal nociceptive system. The fibres linked to nociception (C and A delta) are found in the pulp in a 3/1 ratio. The stabbing pain is lancinating, linked to A delta fibres, myelinated, with a fast conduction velocity. It is associated with reversible pulpitis. It can show a spontaneous or provoked onset and a subsequent duration when the nociceptive stimulus is applied or withdrawn.

Pigg et al[70] state that the location of pain can be determined precisely in cases of advanced stages of irreversible acute pulpal inflammatory processes, where despite being characterised by spontaneous pain, the reaction of the inflamed pupa to different stimuli is even greater, or in the case of irreversible chronic ones where mild pain occurs during chewing or thermal changes.

Fernández Collazo[71] reports in his studies that provoked pain, which persists five minutes after the stimulus that gave rise to it, coincides with the final stages of reversible processes and with irreversible acute processes, where pulp involvement and the inflammatory reaction are greater. There is no pain relief from analgesic therapy at these stages of the pulp inflammatory state (even when the external stimuli that provoked the inflammatory state have been eliminated). At this stage, in addition to vasodilatation and increased permeability of the vascular membrane, increased hydrostatic pressure and blocked lymphatic drainage, the pain becomes unbearable, is exacerbated by hot food and is only relieved by cold liquids.

The form of pain presentation was measured as intermittent or constant. Thus, patients with intermittent pain predominated in the sample. Patients with intermittent pain responded better to treatment than those with constant pain. This behaviour shows that when the pain presented by the patients was intermittent, they responded favourably to treatment.

For Sánchez et al[69] , continuous pain is persistent, intense and dull, linked to amyelinic C-fibres, with slow conduction velocity; it leads to greater suffering and is the one that makes it necessary to seek professional help. It is the typical pain of irreversible pulpitis that denotes greater pulp involvement.

The distance of the lesion to the pulp chamber was measured with a caliper by periapical radiography. Patients who measured the distance of the lesion to the pulp chamber between 2.0mm and 1.5mm responded favourably to treatment with 12 and 9 patients respectively. The closer the lesion was to the pulp chamber, the worse the treatment outcome.

When the caries process reaches the amelodentine boundary, it extends laterally due to the presence of a greater amount of organic tissue at that level.

After spreading along the amelodentine boundary, caries directly attacks the canaliculi in the direction of the pulp. Jolly and Sullivan[67] describe the three-dimensional morphology of caries in detail. The process is initiated by a demineralisation of the dentine, which in turn triggers a defence reaction at the far side of the attack. The progression in dentine takes place at a rate of 180 to 200 um per month. As long as a pulp proximity of 0.75 mm is not reached, no significant pulp reactions will occur. The defence consists of remineralisation or obliteration of the lumen of the canaliculi by a precipitate of calcium salts. If the advance towards the pulp reaches the vicinity of the pulp chamber, tertiary or repair dentine is formed against the advancing lesion. However, if the attack continues unchecked by the defence mechanisms, the acids secreted by the microorganisms eventually demineralise all the mineral substance of the primary, secondary or tertiary dentine and act directly on the pulp tissue, destroying the odontoblasts and forming an abscess.[67]

Bacteria can penetrate up to 0.75 mm of the pulp without causing pulp pathology, but beyond this distance and as they advance, pulp reactions become more intense. Bacterial toxins destroy first the cytoplasm or the fibril of Tomes and then the walls of the canal walls themselves until they disappear. [67]

When the dentine structure gives way, detachments or fissures are produced in the tissue containing necrotic organic remains and bacterial masses that gradually disfigure the constitution of the tooth. The attack of bacterial plaque is not equal over the entire surface, but for various reasons it is concentrated in certain points and advances more rapidly there.[67]

The optical changes observed in an attrition cut are due to the tooth losing minerals during the attack. The depth of demineralisation can be 1 mm below a carious lesion on the surface. Brannstróm et al. produced experimental lesions on permanent human teeth implanted in artificial dentures and observed the following characteristics. Lesions reaching the amelodentine border extended and formed the typical penetration core. In some cases, the underlying dentine was demineralised even if there was a caries cavity in the enamel. Some bacteria were observed in the dentine, the colour of which was brown. Some tubules showed loss of peritubular dentine at an early stage. The intertubular dentine was not demineralised. When the carious cavity reached the dentine, large numbers of bacilli cocci were seen throughout the affected area to great depth along the amelodentine boundary. As dentine demineralisation progressed, the peritubular dentine disappeared completely and bacteria invaded the intertubular dentine. In these areas, the intertubular dentine was relatively dense and contained rounded bodies, with the absence of the fibrillar weft. High mineralisation was observed, especially in the tubules closest to the pulp.

According to Cohen, this is the warning sign that the organism has been attacked and the pulp has reached its physiological tolerance limit, and in this case conservative treatment is necessary. In most cases, a simple removal of the decayed tissue and adequate protection will solve the clinical picture of pain. The pulp always reacts to pain in the same way. Pain is a sensory and emotional experience, not a pleasurable one, with actual or potential tissue damage and serves as an element of anamnesis.

The satisfactory clinical progression of the patients allowed the effectiveness of the treatment to be proven, manifesting in the remission of signs and symptoms of the disease.

Treatment progress was considered favourable when the symptoms had completely subsided 96 hours after treatment. Of the total number of patients, 25 showed a favourable evolution of the treatment. This shows that the sooner the patient comes for consultation, the more effective the treatment will be.

## Conclusions:

- The study found that the most affected age groups were 21 - 25 and 26 - 30 years old and female.
- According to pain intensity, mild pain predominated.
- According to the nature of the pain in the sample, patients with stimulus-induced pain predominated.
- The sample was dominated by patients with intermittent pain.
- Of the total number of patients, the majority had a favourable treatment outcome.
- Patients with mild pain all responded favourably to treatment.
- Patients with provoked and intermittent pain responded more favourably to treatment.
- Patients who measured the distance from the lesion to the pulp chamber as being between 2.0mm and 1.5mm responded favourably to treatment overall.

## Bibliography:


1. Shaffer W, Hine M, Levy B and Tomich C. A Treatise on Oral Pathology. 4th edition. Mexico: Interamericana S.A.; 2018.
2. Khedmat S, Shokouhinejad N. Comparison of the efficacy of three chelating agents in smear layer removal. J Endod. 2018; 34:599-602.
3. Seltzer S, Bender I and Nazimor H. Differential diagnosis of pulp conditions. Oral Surgery, Oral Medicine, Oral Pathology. 2019;19(3):383-91.
4. Robinson and Boling.Dental caries and pulp conditions. 2017; 24:203.
5. Brännström M and Lind P. Pulpal Response to Early Dental Caries. Journal Dental Research. 2018;44(5):1045-50.
6. Kakehashi S, Stanley H and Fitzgerald R. The effects of surgical exposure of dental pulps in germ-free and conventional laboratory rats. Oral Surgery, Oral Medicine, OralPathology. 2017;20(3):340-9.
7. Lasala A. Endodontics. 5th edition. //////:SalvatEditores S.A. 2018.
8. Baume L. Diagnosis of disease of the pulp. Oral Surgery. 2019:29(1):102-16.
9. Calt S, Serper A. Smear layer removal by EGTA. J. Endodon. 2016;26(8):459-61.
10. Mendiburu-Zavala C, Rodríguez-Fernández M. Pulpalpulpary disease in geriatric patients: Prevalence and causes. Latin American Dental Journal (Internet). 2015(Accessed: November 2022);0(2):24-28. Available at:http://www.odontología.uday.mx/revistas/rol/pdf/VOON2p24.pdf.
11. Samra de Quintero P, Rivera-Fuenmayor N. Epidemiology of dental emergencies in children attended at the Faculty of Dentistry of the University of Zulia. CienciaOdontológica 2018;5(2):134-144.
12. Nallian R, Veeratrishul A, Satheesh E Nadeem K, Praveenkumar G Veerasathpurush A. Hospital Emergency Department Visits Attributed to Pulpal and Periapical Disease in the United States in 2016.JOE. 2017:37(1):7-9.
13. Rodríguez-González Y, Ureña-Espinosa M, Portelles-Morales T.

    Clinical and epidemiological behaviour of irreversible pulpitis as a stomatological emergency caused by dental caries. Cuban Society of Stomatology. 2018.
14. León, A. V. Characteristics of pulparee pathologies. Cienfuegos2018:6-8.
15. Parejo, García, Montoro, Herrero, Mayán. Behaviour of the pulp and paediatric diseases in the "Arides Estevez" School, Havana, 2017.

16. Embryology, histology, physiology, pulpal and periapical anatomy, 2022(Accessed: November 2022);Available at: https://dentalexperience.es.tl/EMBRIOLOGIA%2C- HISTOLOGY%2C-PULPAL AND PERIAPICAL-PULPAL-ANATOMY-ANATOMY.htm

17. Kenneth M, Hargreaves. Louis H, Berman. Stephen Cohen. Pulp Histology and Physiology. Universidad del Valle de Atemajac, 2022(Accessed: November 2022). Available at: https://www.studocu.com/es-mx/document/universidad-del-valle- de-atemajac/odontologia/histologia-y-physiologia-pulpar-resumen/14011668

18. Dentin-pulp complex. Structure and diagnosis Abreu Correa Revista de Medicina Isla de la Juventud, 2019(Accessed: November 2022). Available at: https://remij.sld.cu/index.php/remij/article/view/9/22

19. Dentistry Blog: News and articles. Dental pulp characteristics and functionsAdeslasDental_files, 2022(Accessed: November 2022). Available at: https://www.adeslasdental.es/pulpa-del-diente/

20. MsC. Reyes, Oscar Rodríguez. MsC. García Cabrera, Lizet. MsC. Bosch Núñez, Ana Ibis and MsC. Fisiopatología del dolor bucodental: una visiónactualizada del tema. University of Medical Sciences, Faculty of Stomatology, Santiago de Cuba. MEDISAN. 2018;17(9):p 50-8.

21. Oral Health Programme. Health Promotion Service. Canary Islands Health Service. DIRECCIÓN GENERAL DE SALUD PÚBLICA, 2018(Accessed: November 2022). Available in:

https://www3.gobiernodecanarias.org/sanidad/scs/content/b94f644c-5c24-11df-8125- 5700e6e02e85/dolordental.pdf

22. Clínica Gallego, Types of Dental Pain, 2022(Accessed: November 2022) Available at: https://www.clinicagallego.com/noticias/tipos-dolor-dientes/

23. Hennessy, Bernard J. DDS, Texas A&M University, College of DentistryModification/complete review. Toothache(Internet). 2023(Accessed: November 2022). Available at: https://www.merckmanuals.com/es-us/home/buccal-and-dental-disorders/s%C3%ADntoms-of-oral-and-dental-disorders/toothache.

24. SerentilBernaus, Noemi What is dental pain? What can cause dental pain? 2017. Available at: https ://www.propdental. es/dolor-dental/

25. MEDISAN vol.17 no.9 Santiago de Cuba set. 2018. Available at: https://www.google.com/url?sa=t&rct=j&q=&esrc=s&source=web&cd=&ved=2a hUKE

wj2tpmvzczcD9AhUdmGoFHXvOCkEQFnoECCUQAQ&url=https%3A%2F%2Frepository.uft.cl%2Fxmlui%2Fbitstream%2Fhandle%2F20.500.12254%2F557%2FBARAYO N-

BUCAREY%25202017.pdf%3Fsequence%3D1 %26isAllowed%3Dy&usg=AOvVaw3 mbvNwwTX8B0FDjPaoCZGC

26. Socorro Mendiburu Zavala, Celia Elena del Perpetuo. Peñaloza Cuevas, Ricardo. Chuc Baas, Inés del Rosario. Medina Peralta, Salvador. Rev CubanaEstomatol. jul.-set. 2017(Cited Oct. 2022);54(3): [approx 5 pp]. Available from: http://scielo.sld.cu/scielo.php?script=sci arttext&pid=S0034-75072017000300004

27. Types of dental pulp diseases. (Cited October 2022);Available at: https://estudidentalbarcelona.com/tipos-enfermedades-la-pulpa-dental/

28. Rebel, Serper A. Smear layer removal by EGTA.2013;26(8):459-61.

29. Seltzer Samuel, Bender J.B. Dental Pulp. 9th edition: Editorial Manual Moderno; 2014. p 43.

30. Bakland LK, Grossman. Endodontics. 4th Edition. Mexico. Editorial McGraw-Hill Interamericana, 2015.

31. Morse, Chen, M.; R.M. Andersen: Comparing Oral Health Care Systems, WHO, Geneva. 2014,213:6.

32. Soberaniz-Morales V, Alonzo-Echeverría L, Vega-Lizama EM. Frequency of pulp and paper pathology in the hospital clinic of petróleosmexicanos Coatzacoalcos, Veracruz. Rev CienOdontol. 2015;8(1):7-12.

33. Duque de Estrada RiverónJohany, Pérez Quiñónez José Alberto, Hidalgo-Gato Fuentes Iliana. Dental caries and oral ecology, important aspects to consider. Rev. CubanaEstomatol(Internet). 2014(cited 8 May 2021):43(1): [Approx. 8 pp]. Available from: http://scielo.sld.cu/

34. Nyerere JW, Matee MI, Simon ENM. Emergency pulpotomy in relieving acute dental pain among Tanzanian patients.BMC Oral Health.;2018:6:1.

35. González Naya G, Montero del Castillo ME. Comprehensive General Stomatology. Havana: CienciasMédicas; 2013. P 78.

36. Lanziano Lobo, María José. Parra Hernández, Silvia Nathalia. Jiménez Manrique, Raúl Andrés. University Santo Tomas, Bucaramanga. Health Sciences Division. Faculty of Dentistry. Pulpal and periapical pathologies. 2020(cited 25 May 2021). Available at: https://repository.usta.edu.co/bitstream/handle/11634/30825/2020LanzianoMaria.pdi2se quence=9&isAllowed=y

37. Hennessy, Bernard J. DDS, Texas A&M University, College of Dentistry. Pulpitis. Mar. 2021(cited 8 May 2021). Available from:

https: //www. msdmanuals .com/pro fes sional/trastornos - odontol%C3%B3gicos/trastornos-odontol%C3%B3gicos-comunes/pulpitis

38. Arias, Estela. Reversible or Irreversible Pulpitis: symptoms and treatment. Dec. 2022(cited 8 May 2021). Available at: https://www.smysecret.com/blog/general/pulpitis- reversible-o-irreversible/

39. Clínica Dental Ruiz de Gopegui What is reversible pulpitis? Mar-2022(cited 8 May 2021) Available at: https://www.clinicaruizdegopegui.com/pulpitis-reversibles/

40. Causes and treatment of pulpitis. Sanitas.es. 2023(cited 8 May 2021). Available at: https://www/%20y%20tratamiento%20de%20la%20pulpitis.htm

41. Cuba-Cueto, Karla Samanta. VillavicencioCaparó, Ebingen. Perfilepidemiológico de patologíaspulpares y periapicalesenLatinoamérica, agosto 2022 (cited 8 May 2021). Available at: https://revistas.ug.edu.ec/index.php/eoug/article/view/1424/2446

42. Areas Cruz, Estela. Reversible or Irreversible Pulpitis: symptoms and treatment. December 2022(cited 8 May 2021). Available at: https://www.smysecret.com/blog/general/pulpitis-reversible-o-irreversible/

43. Pérez, Belén. Clínica dental Getxo. What is reversible pulpitis? February 2022(cited 8 May 2021). Available at: https://belenperezdental.com/pulpitis-reversible/

44. Estudi Dental Barcelona: What is reversible pulpitis and what is its treatment? November 2017(cited 8 May 2021). Available at: https://estudidentalbarcelona.com/la-pulpitis-reversible-tratamiento/

45. Ibi Dental Clinic. Reversible pulpitis and irreversible pulpitis. July 2017(cited 8 May 2021). Available at: https://www.clinicacimeribi.com/pulpitis/

46. Hennessy Bernard J. DDS, Texas A&M University, College of Dentistry, Medically Reviewed. Pulpitis. Mar. 2021(cited 8 May 2021). Available at: https ://www. msdmanuals .com/pro fes sional/trastornos - odontol%C3%B3gicos/trastornos-odontol%C3%B3gicos-comunes/pulpitis.

47. Dr. de la Cruz, Javier. Reversible pulpitis: what it is and how to treat it. March, 2022. (cited 8 May 2022). Available at: https://www.bordonclinic.com/pulpitis-reversible-que-es-y- como-tratarla/.

48. IOM Dental, Endodontics, General Dentistry, Treatment of reversible pulpitis. 2019(cited 8 May 2021). Available from: https://iomdental.es/blog/tratamiento-de-la- pulpitis-reversible/

49. Dr. Pardiñas López, Simón, What is pulpitis and how is it treated? 2022. Available at: https://gacetadental.com/2022/11/que-es-la-pulpitis-y-como-se-trata-37885/
50. Revista Cubana de Estomatología. Oct-Dec 2018(cited 8 May 2021);49(4): [Approx. 8 pp.] Available from:http://scielo.sld.cu/scielo.php?script=sci arttext&pid=S0034- 75072012000400004
51. Treatment of pulpitis. Sanitas.es. 2023. (cited 8 May 2021). Available at: https://www.sanitas.es/sanitas/seguros/es/particulares/biblioteca-de-salud/salud-dental/caries-empastes/pulpitis.html.
52. Clinical diagnostic guide for pulpal and periapical pathologies. Adapted and updated version of the consensus conference recommended diagnostic terminology, American Association of Endodontics, 2017. (cited 8 May 2021) Available at: https://www.iztacala.unam.mx/rrivas/notas/notas7patpulpar/revdefLnicion.html
53. 53.Abreu, René. Reversible Pulpitis: A Dental Discomfort. 2022. Rev. Odontol. 2022(cited 8 May 2021);vol5(7):[approx 5 pp.] Available from: https://www.odonton.es/pulpitis-reversible-una-molestia-dental/
54. Villasana, Arelys. PatologíaPulpar y suDiagnóstico. Venezuela: Universidad Central de Venezuela, 2018.
55. Author and Title. Rev CubanaEstomatol.May-Aug 2017 (cited 8 May 2021);39(2): [approx 6 pp]. Available from: http://scielo.sld.cu/scielo.php?script=sci arttext&pid=S0034-75072002000200005
56. González Escobar, Raimara. Pharmaceutical Information Centre. Eugenol: pharmacological and toxicological properties. Advantages and disadvantages of its use. RevistaCubana de Estomatología. August 2019(cited 8 May 2021). Available at: https ://pesquisa.bvsalud. org/portal/resource/pt/lil-351649
57. Pérez Martínez, Aarón. Guerrero Ibarra, Jorge. Celis Rivas, Luis. Effect of residual eugenol in root canals on the adhesion of prefabricated luminescent endoprostheses cemented with composite resinRev. Odont. Mex. Jan./Mar.2016(cited 8 May 2021);18(1): [approx 6 pp]. Available from: https://www.scielo.org.mx/scielo.php?script=sci arttext&pid=S1870-199X2014000100003
58. Guzman JRM, Pantoja GV Eugenol: dental material with risk of local and systemic toxicity. Available at:https://www.medigraphic.com/cgi-bin/new/resumen.cgi?IDARTICULO=26021
59. Katz J, Melzack R. Measurement of pain. SurgClin North Am. 1999; 79:231-52.
60. Jiménez Zúñiga Luis A. Pulpal pain. Anatomophysiological considerations.

Universidad Central de Venezuela[Internet]. 2014: [cited19April 2021]. Available from: http://www.carlosbóveda.com/ odontolofolder/ odontologoinvitado 41htm.

61. RuizdeGopegui,J.,H. Fabra. Endodontic failure without apparent cause. Rev Endodontics. 2017:20(4):250-7.

62. Zúñiga Delgado A, Gaviria Delgado, AS. Prevalence of pulpal lesions in patients treated with Endodontics in the clinic. Odontologic School of the University of Valle. Colombian Rev. 2016:12.

63. Portal Macías LG. Behaviour of the stomatological emergency service at the "Pedro Celestino Aguilera González" clinic in the municipality of Playa. RevHabCienciasMéd [Internet]. 2018 [citedApr 2022]; 12(1): [approx. 10 p.]. Available from: http://www.bvs.sld.cu/revistas/rhab/vol 12 1 13/rhcm10113.htm.

64. Fernández Cortina TJ. Pulpal pathologies and primary endodontic treatments. Case study. Central University of Venezuela. Faculty of Stomatology. [Internet]. 2015[citedMarch 2018];171. Available from: http ://saber.ucv. ve/jspui/handle/123456789/4054\.

65. Quiñonez D. Pulpal and periapical pathologies most frequently encountered in 2 stomatological clinics. Rev CubanaEstomatol, 2016:37 (2):84-88.

66. Boltacz-Rzepkowska E, Laszkiewicz J. Endodontic treatment and periapical health in patients of the Institute of Dentistry in Lodz.Przegl Epidemiol;2017: 59(1):107-15.

67. Julio Barrancos M. Dental histopathology. In: Operatoria Dental: Editorial Médica Panamericana, 1999.p 260-262.

68. Pérez Ruíz AO, Ventura Hernández MI, Valverde Grandal O. Description of the functional properties of the trigeminal muciceptive system in relation to pulpal pain. RevCubEstomatol [Internet]. 2015 Jul-Sep [citedApr 2022]; 52(3): [approx. 15 p.].

Available at: http://www.revestomatologia.sld.cu/ index.php/est/article/view/376/199

69. Sánchez Rodríguez R, Souto Román MC, Rosales Corría EN, PardíasMilán LC, Guerra López AM. Oral diseases that constitute stomatological emergencies.

MULTIMED [Internet]. 2015 [citedApr 2018]; 19(3): [approx. 16 p.]. Available from: http://www.medigraphic.com/pdfs/multimed/mul-2015/mul153p.pdf.

70. Pigg M, Svensson P, Drangsholt M, List T. Seven-year follow-up of patients diagnosed with atypical odontalgia: A prospective study. J Orofac Pain [Internet]. 2016;27(2):151- 64.

71. Montoro Ferrer Y, Fernández Collazo ME. Stomatological emergencies due to pulp

lesions. Rev. CubanaEstomatología. Ciudad de La Habana. Oct-Dec. 2019;49(4):

Annexes:

Annex 2: Form:

- Name:
- Age: Sex:
- History of the disease

current:

---

1- Intensity of pain

Mild

Moderate

__ Intense

2- Nature of pain.

Provoked

__ Spontaneous

3- Form of presentation of pain.

Constant

__ Intermittent

4- Depth of injury:

0.5 mm

1.0 mm

1.5 mm

2.0 mm

5- Pain remission time:

96 h ______No referral.

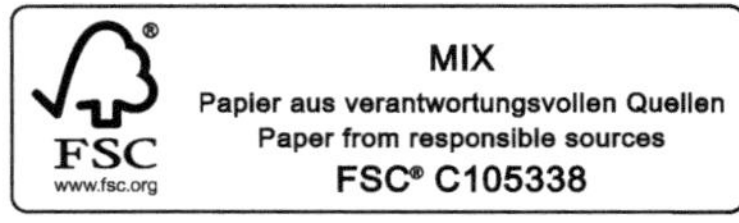


Printed by Books on Demand GmbH, Norderstedt / Germany